Low nickel diet cookbook 2024

Nourishing Creations: Elevate Your Low Nickel Diet with Inspired Culinary Innovations

Elsie J. Smith

Table of Contents

Introduction to a Low Nickel Diet

Emma had always enjoyed experimenting in the kitchen, creating delicious meals for her family and friends. But when she started experiencing persistent rashes, digestive issues, and unexplained fatigue, she knew something had to change. After numerous doctor visits and tests, Emma was diagnosed with a nickel allergy. The news was overwhelming, and she struggled to find reliable information on how to manage her condition through diet.

One evening, while researching online, Emma discovered the "Low Nickel Diet Cookbook 2024." The book promised not only a collection of low nickel recipes but also a comprehensive guide to understanding and managing a nickel allergy. Hopeful and eager for a solution, she decided to purchase the cookbook.

When the cookbook arrived, Emma was immediately impressed by its thorough introduction to nickel sensitivity. It explained the symptoms, diagnosis, and the significant impact a low nickel diet could have on her overall health. The detailed guidelines on foods to avoid and safe alternatives were a game-changer for Emma, who had felt lost trying to navigate her new dietary restrictions.

Emma started her mornings with the cookbook's breakfast recipes, transforming her usual routine. The "Fluffy Rice Flour

Pancakes" became a favorite, offering a delicious, nickel-free start to her day. The "Banana and Blueberry Smoothie" was another hit, providing a refreshing and nutritious option that kept her energized.

Lunchtime, once a challenge, became a delight with recipes like the "Grilled Chicken and Rice Salad" and "Tuna and Avocado Lettuce Wraps." These meals were not only safe for her to eat but also bursting with flavor, proving that a low nickel diet didn't mean compromising on taste. Emma enjoyed experimenting with the variety of salads and soups, each recipe contributing to her newfound sense of wellness.

Dinners, which used to be a source of stress, were now an opportunity for Emma to explore new culinary horizons. The "Baked Lemon Herb Fish" was a regular feature at her dinner table, impressing her family with its simplicity and flavor. The "Beef and Vegetable Stir-Fry" offered a quick and satisfying meal after long days, and the "Chicken and Rice Casserole" became a comforting favorite.

The cookbook didn't stop at main meals; it also provided Emma with creative snack and side options. She loved the "Cottage Cheese and Cucumber Salad" for its light and refreshing taste, perfect for mid-afternoon hunger pangs. The desserts, such as the "Fruit-Based Sweet Treats," allowed her to indulge without worrying about nickel content, bringing back the joy of guilt-free eating.

As Emma followed the meal plans and tips for dining out, she noticed significant improvements in her health. The rashes faded, her digestion improved, and her energy levels soared. The cookbook's practical advice on grocery shopping and meal prep made adhering to a low nickel diet manageable and sustainable, even on her busiest days.

Emma's transformation didn't go unnoticed. Her friends and family were curious about her newfound vitality and the delicious meals she was creating. She eagerly shared her story and recommended the "Low Nickel Diet Cookbook 2024" to anyone struggling with similar issues. For Emma, the cookbook was more than just a collection of recipes; it was a lifeline, offering hope, guidance, and a path to better health.

So, why should someone buy the "Low Nickel Diet Cookbook 2024"? Because it's a comprehensive resource that demystifies the complexities of a low nickel diet. It provides not only a wide array of delicious, safe recipes but also the knowledge and tools needed to manage nickel sensitivity effectively. For anyone seeking to improve their health and enjoy their meals without worry, this cookbook is an invaluable guide to a happier, healthier life.

What is Nickel Allergy?

Nickel allergy is a common condition affecting a significant portion of the population, characterized by an adverse reaction to nickel exposure. Nickel is a metal found in various everyday items, including jewelry, coins, and even some foods. For those with a nickel allergy, contact with nickel can trigger symptoms ranging from mild skin irritation to severe systemic reactions. This condition can be particularly challenging to manage because nickel is so prevalent in our environment and diet.

When someone with a nickel allergy is exposed to the metal, their immune system mistakenly identifies nickel as a harmful substance. This leads to an allergic reaction, typically manifesting as contact dermatitis. Symptoms often include redness, itching, swelling, and the development of small blisters at the site of contact. While contact dermatitis is the most common symptom, some individuals may also experience more severe reactions, such as gastrointestinal distress when ingesting nickel through food.

Managing a nickel allergy often involves significant lifestyle adjustments, particularly concerning diet. Nickel can be found in many foods, including nuts, seeds, chocolate, certain fruits and vegetables, and even grains. For those with a severe allergy, even small amounts of dietary nickel can trigger reactions. Therefore, adhering to a low nickel diet is crucial to minimize exposure and alleviate symptoms.

The "Low Nickel Diet Cookbook 2024" serves as an essential resource for individuals diagnosed with nickel allergy. It provides comprehensive guidance on avoiding high-nickel foods and substituting them with safer alternatives. By following the dietary recommendations and recipes in the cookbook, individuals can significantly reduce their nickel intake, leading to fewer allergic reactions and an overall improvement in quality of life.

Understanding the sources of dietary nickel is fundamental for managing this allergy. Foods such as legumes, nuts, and whole grains, which are typically considered healthy, can be problematic for those with a nickel allergy. The cookbook offers practical solutions by suggesting low-nickel substitutes that still provide the necessary nutrients without triggering allergic reactions. This allows individuals to maintain a balanced and nutritious diet without compromising their health.

In addition to dietary changes, the cookbook emphasizes the importance of proper food preparation and cooking methods to reduce nickel content. For example, cooking with stainless steel pots and pans can leach nickel into food, exacerbating symptoms. The cookbook provides tips on using nickel-free cookware and other kitchen tools to further minimize exposure. These practical insights help individuals create a safe cooking environment, making the management of their allergy more feasible.

By following the guidelines and recipes in the "Low Nickel Diet Cookbook 2024," individuals with a nickel allergy can take control of their health and well-being. The cookbook empowers them with the knowledge and tools needed to navigate their dietary restrictions confidently. With careful planning and the right resources, living with a nickel allergy becomes manageable, allowing individuals to enjoy a diverse and satisfying diet while minimizing their symptoms and improving their overall health.

Symptoms and Diagnosis

Nickel allergy, often manifesting through contact dermatitis, can also impact those sensitive to ingested nickel. The symptoms can vary widely and often resemble other allergic reactions, making diagnosis challenging. Common symptoms include persistent itching, redness, and rashes, typically occurring at points of contact with nickel-containing items like jewelry, belt buckles, or even mobile phones. These skin reactions can spread to other areas, becoming more severe with prolonged exposure.

Ingested nickel can cause gastrointestinal issues such as nausea, vomiting, and abdominal pain. Some individuals may experience headaches, chronic fatigue, or a general sense of malaise. The connection between these symptoms and nickel sensitivity is often overlooked, as they can be mistaken for other dietary intolerances or health conditions. This makes awareness and proper diagnosis critical for effective management.

Identifying a nickel allergy typically begins with a detailed medical history and physical examination. Dermatologists often use patch testing, where small amounts of nickel are applied to the skin under adhesive patches. These patches are left in place for 48 hours, and the skin is then examined for any allergic reactions.

Positive reactions, such as redness, itching, or blistering at the test site, indicate a nickel allergy.

For those suspecting a dietary nickel sensitivity, elimination diets can be particularly revealing. Under medical supervision, individuals remove high-nickel foods from their diet for a period, monitoring symptom changes. Common high-nickel foods include nuts, chocolate, legumes, and certain grains. After the elimination phase, foods are gradually reintroduced to identify specific triggers. This method helps confirm the link between dietary nickel and symptoms, guiding dietary adjustments.

Blood tests may also be employed, though they are less definitive for nickel allergies compared to patch testing. Elevated levels of nickel in the blood or abnormal immune responses to nickel can support the diagnosis, especially when combined with clinical symptoms and history. However, these tests are often supplementary, used to provide additional confirmation rather than primary diagnosis.

Once diagnosed, managing nickel allergy involves both avoiding contact with nickel-containing items and adhering to a low-nickel diet. The "Low Nickel Diet Cookbook 2024" serves as a crucial tool in this regard, offering recipes and dietary guidance to minimize nickel intake while ensuring nutritional balance. This approach not only alleviates symptoms but also supports overall health and well-being, making dietary management practical and enjoyable.

In summary, recognizing and diagnosing nickel allergy is a multifaceted process, involving a combination of medical history, physical examination, patch testing, elimination diets, and sometimes blood tests. Understanding the symptoms and undergoing proper diagnostic procedures is essential for effective management. The "Low Nickel Diet Cookbook 2024" provides a comprehensive resource for those diagnosed with nickel allergy, helping them navigate their dietary restrictions with ease and confidence, ultimately leading to improved health and quality of life.

Benefits of a Low Nickel Diet

Following a low nickel diet can significantly enhance the quality of life for individuals with nickel sensitivity or allergy. Nickel, a common element found in many foods and everyday items, can trigger various adverse reactions in sensitive individuals. By adhering to a low nickel diet, individuals can effectively manage and mitigate symptoms such as skin rashes, itching, gastrointestinal distress, and fatigue, leading to a noticeable improvement in their overall well-being.

One of the primary benefits of a low nickel diet is the reduction of dermatitis, particularly hand eczema, which is a common reaction among those with nickel allergy. Consuming high-nickel foods can exacerbate skin conditions, causing discomfort and persistent itching. The "Low Nickel Diet Cookbook 2024" provides recipes and meal plans that avoid high-nickel ingredients, helping individuals maintain clear, healthy skin and avoid flare-ups that disrupt daily activities and quality of life.

Digestive health also sees marked improvement with a low nickel diet. Nickel sensitivity can lead to gastrointestinal issues such as nausea, abdominal pain, and bloating. By eliminating foods high in nickel and focusing on safe alternatives, individuals can alleviate these uncomfortable symptoms. The cookbook offers a variety of delicious, low-nickel recipes that support digestive health while ensuring balanced nutrition and satisfying meals.

Energy levels are another area where individuals may notice significant benefits. Nickel exposure can lead to chronic fatigue, making it difficult to maintain energy throughout the day. By following a diet that minimizes nickel intake, individuals often experience increased energy levels and reduced fatigue. The nutritious and varied recipes in the "Low Nickel Diet Cookbook 2024" provide the necessary fuel to keep energy levels stable, supporting an active and fulfilling lifestyle.

In addition to physical health improvements, a low nickel diet can enhance mental well-being. The constant discomfort and unpredictability of nickel allergy symptoms can lead to stress and anxiety. Adopting a low nickel diet and having a reliable resource like the cookbook to guide meal choices can provide peace of mind, reducing anxiety and stress associated with managing the condition. Knowing that each meal is safe and nutritious helps build confidence and a positive outlook.

Nutritional balance is another key benefit of the low nickel diet as outlined in the cookbook. The carefully crafted recipes ensure that individuals do not miss out on essential nutrients while avoiding high-nickel foods. The cookbook emphasizes the inclusion of a wide variety of low-nickel ingredients that provide a well-rounded diet, promoting overall health and preventing nutritional deficiencies that can arise from dietary restrictions.

Finally, the "Low Nickel Diet Cookbook 2024" fosters a sense of culinary enjoyment and creativity. It demonstrates that a low nickel diet does not have to be monotonous or bland. With inventive and tasty recipes, individuals can explore new flavors and cooking techniques, making mealtime an enjoyable and adventurous experience. This positive relationship with food enhances adherence to the diet and encourages long-term commitment to healthy eating habits.

Overall, the benefits of a low nickel diet are vast and impactful, addressing both physical and mental health concerns. The "Low Nickel Diet Cookbook 2024" is an essential tool for anyone looking to improve their health and manage nickel sensitivity through informed and enjoyable dietary choices. By offering practical, delicious, and nutritionally balanced recipes, the cookbook empowers individuals to lead healthier, happier lives free from the burdens of nickel allergy symptoms.

Chapter 1: Breakfast Recipes

Fluffy Rice Flour Pancakes

Ingredient:

- 1 cup rice flour
- 2 tablespoons sugar
- 1 tablespoon baking powder
- 1/2 teaspoon salt
- 1 cup rice milk
- 2 tablespoons vegetable oil (low-nickel option like canola oil)
- 1 egg
- 1 teaspoon vanilla extract

Instructions:

1. In a large bowl, combine rice flour, sugar, baking powder, and salt.

2. In another bowl, whisk together rice milk, vegetable oil, egg, and vanilla extract.

3. Pour the wet ingredients into the dry ingredients and mix until just combined. Be careful not to overmix; the batter should be slightly lumpy.

4. Heat a non-stick skillet or griddle over medium heat and lightly grease it with a small amount of oil.

5. Pour 1/4 cup of batter onto the skillet for each pancake. Cook until bubbles form on the surface and the edges look set, about 2-3 minutes.

6. Flip the pancakes and cook for an additional 2-3 minutes, until golden brown and cooked through.

7. Serve warm with your choice of low-nickel toppings, such as fresh fruit, pure maple syrup, or a dollop of rice-based whipped cream.

Nutritional Information:

- Calories: 190 per serving
- Protein: 3g
- Carbohydrates: 32g
- Fat: 5g
- Fiber: 1g

Serving Size:

4 pancakes

Cooking Time:

15 minutes

Creamy Rice Porridge with Cinnamon

Ingredient:

1 cup white rice

4 cups water

1 cup rice milk

1 teaspoon ground cinnamon

1 tablespoon honey (optional)

1/4 teaspoon salt

Instructions:

1. Rinse the rice under cold water until the water runs clear.

2. In a medium saucepan, combine the rinsed rice and water. Bring to a boil over medium-high heat.

3. Once boiling, reduce the heat to low, cover, and simmer for 20 minutes or until the rice is tender and the water is absorbed.

4. Add the rice milk, cinnamon, honey (if using), and salt to the cooked rice. Stir well to combine.

5. Cook over low heat, stirring frequently, for an additional 10 minutes until the porridge reaches a creamy consistency.

6. Remove from heat and let sit for a few minutes before serving.

Nutritional Information:

Calories: 180 per serving

Protein: 3g

Carbohydrates: 38g

Fat: 2g

Fiber: 1g

Serving Size:

4 servings

Cooking Time:

30 minutes

Banana and Blueberry Smoothie

Ingredient:

- 1 ripe banana
- 1/2 cup fresh blueberries
- 1 cup almond milk
- 1 tablespoon honey (optional)
- 1/2 cup ice cubes

Instructions:

1. Place the banana, blueberries, almond milk, honey (if using), and ice cubes in a blender.
2. Blend on high until smooth and creamy.
3. Serve immediately for the best flavor and texture.

Nutritional Information:

- Calories: 180
- Protein: 2g
- Carbohydrates: 44g
- Fat: 1.5g
- Fiber: 4g

Serving Size:

1 serving (approximately 1.5 cups)

Cooking Time:

5 minutes

Egg and Vegetable Frittata

Ingredient:

- 6 large eggs
- 1/2 cup milk
- 1 cup chopped spinach
- 1/2 cup diced bell peppers (red or yellow)
- 1/4 cup diced onions
- 2 tablespoons olive oil
- Salt and pepper to taste

Instructions:

1. Preheat the oven to 375°F (190°C).
2. In a large mixing bowl, whisk together eggs and milk until well combined. Season with salt and pepper.
3. Heat olive oil in a 10-inch oven-safe skillet over medium heat. Add onions and bell peppers, sautéing until vegetables are soft, about 5 minutes.
4. Add spinach to the skillet and cook until just wilted.
5. Pour the egg mixture over the vegetables, stirring slightly to ensure even distribution.

6. Cook without stirring for about 2 minutes until the edges begin to set.

7. Transfer the skillet to the preheated oven and bake for 15-18 minutes, or until the frittata is set and lightly golden on top.

8. Remove from the oven and let cool for a few minutes before slicing and serving.

Nutritional Information:

- Calories: 150 per serving
- Protein: 9g
- Carbohydrates: 4g
- Fat: 11g
- Fiber: 1g

Serving Size:

Serves 4

Cooking Time:

Approximately 25-30 minutes (including preparation and baking)

Gluten-Free Muffins

Ingredient:

- 2 cups gluten-free flour blend
- 1 teaspoon baking powder
- 1/2 teaspoon baking soda
- 1/4 teaspoon salt
- 1/2 cup unsalted butter, softened
- 3/4 cup sugar
- 2 large eggs
- 1 teaspoon vanilla extract
- 1 cup milk (or non-dairy alternative)
- 1 cup blueberries (fresh or frozen)

Instructions:

1. Preheat the oven to 375°F (190°C).
2. Line a muffin tin with paper liners or grease with non-stick spray.
3. In a medium bowl, whisk together gluten-free flour, baking powder, baking soda, and salt.
4. In a large bowl, cream the butter and sugar until light and fluffy.
5. Beat in the eggs one at a time, then stir in the vanilla extract.

6. Alternately add the flour mixture and milk to the butter mixture, starting and ending with the flour.

7. Gently fold in the blueberries.

8. Spoon the batter into the prepared muffin tin, filling each cup about two-thirds full.

9. Bake for 20-25 minutes, or until a toothpick inserted into the center of a muffin comes out clean.

10. Allow to cool in the pan for 5 minutes before transferring to a wire rack to cool completely.

Nutritional Information:

- Calories: 210
- Protein: 4g
- Carbohydrates: 32g
- Fat: 8g
- Fiber: 2g

Serving Size:

1 muffin

Cooking Time:

25 minutes

Ingredient List:

- 1 cup rice milk
- 1 cup mixed berries (such as strawberries, blueberries, and raspberries)
- 1/2 cup gluten-free granola
- 2 tablespoons honey
- 1 teaspoon vanilla extract

Instructions:

1. In a small bowl, combine rice milk and vanilla extract.
2. In serving glasses, layer half of the granola at the bottom.
3. Add a layer of mixed berries over the granola.
4. Drizzle a tablespoon of honey over the berries.
5. Pour half of the rice milk mixture evenly over the first set of layers.
6. Repeat the layering process with the remaining granola, berries, honey, and rice milk.
7. Chill in the refrigerator for at least 30 minutes before serving to allow the flavors to meld.

Nutritional Information:

- Calories: 270
- Carbohydrates: 49g
- Protein: 4g
- Fat: 6g
- Sodium: 30mg
- Fiber: 4g

Serving Size:

- This recipe serves 2.

Cooking Time:

- Preparation time: 10 minutes
- Chill time: 30 minutes

Quinoa Breakfast Bowl

Ingredients:

- 1 cup quinoa
- 2 cups water
- 1 cup almond milk (or any low-nickel plant-based milk)
- 1 tablespoon honey or maple syrup
- 1 teaspoon vanilla extract
- 1/2 teaspoon ground cinnamon
- 1/4 cup fresh blueberries
- 1/4 cup sliced strawberries
- 1/4 cup chopped walnuts (optional, check for individual nickel tolerance)
- Fresh mint leaves for garnish

Instructions:

1. Rinse the quinoa thoroughly under cold water to remove any saponins.
2. In a medium saucepan, bring the water to a boil. Add the quinoa, reduce heat to low, cover, and simmer for 15 minutes or until the water is absorbed and the quinoa is tender.
3. In a separate small saucepan, heat the almond milk over medium heat until warm but not boiling.

4. Add the cooked quinoa to the warmed almond milk. Stir in the honey (or maple syrup), vanilla extract, and ground cinnamon. Mix well until the quinoa is evenly coated and the mixture is heated through.

5. Remove from heat and divide the quinoa mixture into serving bowls.

6. Top each bowl with fresh blueberries, sliced strawberries, and chopped walnuts, if using.

7. Garnish with fresh mint leaves before serving.

Nutritional Information:

- Calories: 320 per serving
- Protein: 9 grams
- Carbohydrates: 50 grams
- Dietary Fiber: 7 grams
- Sugars: 15 grams
- Fat: 10 grams
- Saturated Fat: 1 gram
- Sodium: 60 milligrams

Serving Size:

- Makes 2 servings

Cooking Time:

- Total time: 30 minutes (Prep time: 5 minutes, Cook time: 25 minutes)

Ingredient:

- 2 large rice cakes
- 1 apple, thinly sliced
- 1 teaspoon ground cinnamon
- 1 tablespoon honey or maple syrup
- 1 tablespoon unsweetened almond butter (optional)
- A pinch of sea salt

Instructions:

1. Toast the rice cakes lightly until they are crisp.
2. Spread a thin layer of unsweetened almond butter on each rice cake if desired.
3. Arrange the thinly sliced apple pieces evenly on top of the rice cakes.
4. Drizzle the honey or maple syrup over the apple slices.
5. Sprinkle the ground cinnamon and a pinch of sea salt over the top.
6. Serve immediately while the rice cakes are still crisp and the apples are fresh.

Nutritional Information:

- Calories: 150 per serving
- Protein: 2g
- Carbohydrates: 30g
- Sugars: 15g
- Fat: 2g
- Fiber: 4g
- Sodium: 50mg

Serving Size: 2 rice cakes

Cooking Time: 10 minutes

Rice Flour Waffles

Ingredients:

- 1 cup rice flour
- 1 tablespoon baking powder
- 1 tablespoon sugar
- 1/4 teaspoon salt
- 1 cup milk (dairy or non-dairy)
- 2 tablespoons vegetable oil
- 1 large egg
- 1 teaspoon vanilla extract

Instructions:

1. Preheat your waffle iron according to the manufacturer's instructions.
2. In a large mixing bowl, combine the rice flour, baking powder, sugar, and salt.
3. In another bowl, whisk together the milk, vegetable oil, egg, and vanilla extract.
4. Pour the wet ingredients into the dry ingredients and mix until just combined. The batter may be slightly lumpy.
5. Lightly grease the waffle iron with oil or non-stick spray.

6. Pour enough batter into the waffle iron to cover the surface, then close and cook according to the waffle iron's instructions, typically for about 4-5 minutes, or until the waffles are golden brown and crisp.

7. Carefully remove the waffles and repeat with the remaining batter.

Nutritional Information:

- Calories: 180 per waffle
- Protein: 4g
- Carbohydrates: 26g
- Dietary Fiber: 1g
- Sugars: 4g
- Fat: 6g
- Saturated Fat: 1g
- Cholesterol: 35mg
- Sodium: 230mg

Serving Size:

- Makes approximately 4 waffles

Cooking Time:

- Preparation Time: 10 minutes
- Cooking Time: 15-20 minutes

Spinach and Feta Omelet

Ingredients:

- 2 large eggs
- 1/2 cup fresh spinach leaves, chopped
- 1/4 cup crumbled feta cheese
- 1 tablespoon olive oil
- Salt and pepper to taste

Instructions:

1. In a bowl, whisk the eggs until they are well combined and slightly frothy. Season with a pinch of salt and pepper.
2. Heat the olive oil in a non-stick skillet over medium heat. Add the chopped spinach and sauté for 2-3 minutes, until wilted.
3. Pour the beaten eggs over the spinach in the skillet. Cook for 2-3 minutes, until the eggs start to set around the edges.
4. Sprinkle the crumbled feta cheese evenly over one half of the omelet.
5. Using a spatula, carefully fold the omelet in half, covering the feta cheese. Cook for another 2 minutes, until the eggs are fully set and the cheese is slightly melted.
6. Slide the omelet onto a plate and serve immediately.

Nutritional Information:

- Calories: 230
- Protein: 15g
- Carbohydrates: 3g
- Fat: 18g
- Fiber: 1g
- Sodium: 350mg

Serving Size: 1 omelet

Cooking Time: 10 minutes

Chapter 2: Lunch Recipes

Grilled Chicken and Rice Salad

Ingredients:

- 2 boneless, skinless chicken breasts
- 1 cup cooked brown rice
- 1 cup chopped romaine lettuce
- 1/2 cup diced cucumber
- 1/2 cup cherry tomatoes, halved
- 1/4 cup shredded carrots
- 1/4 cup sliced red bell pepper
- 2 tablespoons olive oil
- 1 tablespoon lemon juice
- 1 teaspoon dried oregano
- Salt and pepper to taste

Instructions:

1. Preheat the grill to medium-high heat.
2. Season the chicken breasts with salt, pepper, and dried oregano.
3. Grill the chicken for 6-7 minutes on each side, or until fully cooked and no longer pink in the center.

4. Remove the chicken from the grill and let it rest for a few minutes before slicing into thin strips.

5. In a large bowl, combine the cooked brown rice, chopped romaine lettuce, diced cucumber, cherry tomatoes, shredded carrots, and sliced red bell pepper.

6. In a small bowl, whisk together the olive oil and lemon juice.

7. Drizzle the dressing over the salad and toss to combine.

8. Top the salad with the grilled chicken strips.

9. Serve immediately.

Nutritional Information:

- Calories: 350
- Protein: 28g
- Carbohydrates: 25g
- Dietary Fiber: 4g
- Total Fat: 15g
- Saturated Fat: 2.5g
- Cholesterol: 70mg
- Sodium: 150mg

Serving Size:

- Serves 2

Cooking Time:

- 25 minutes

Quinoa and Vegetable Stir-Fry

Ingredients:

- 1 cup quinoa
- 2 cups water or low-sodium vegetable broth
- 1 tablespoon olive oil
- 1 small zucchini, diced
- 1 small yellow squash, diced
- 1 cup cherry tomatoes, halved
- 1/2 cup finely chopped bell pepper
- 1/4 cup chopped fresh parsley
- 1 lemon, juiced
- Salt and pepper to taste

Instructions:

1. Rinse the quinoa under cold water to remove any bitterness. In a medium saucepan, combine the quinoa and water (or vegetable broth) and bring to a boil.
2. Reduce the heat to low, cover, and simmer for about 15 minutes, or until the quinoa is cooked and the liquid is absorbed. Fluff with a fork and set aside.

3. In a large skillet, heat the olive oil over medium heat. Add the diced zucchini and yellow squash, and sauté for about 5 minutes, or until they begin to soften.

4. Add the cherry tomatoes and bell pepper to the skillet, and cook for an additional 3-4 minutes, stirring occasionally.

5. Remove the skillet from the heat and stir in the cooked quinoa and chopped parsley.

6. Drizzle the lemon juice over the mixture and season with salt and pepper to taste. Mix well to combine all the flavors.

7. Serve warm or at room temperature.

Nutritional Information:

- Calories: 250
- Protein: 8g
- Carbohydrates: 40g
- Fiber: 6g
- Fat: 7g
- Sodium: 50mg

Serving Size:

Serves 4

Cooking Time:

25 minutes

Tuna and Avocado Lettuce Wraps

Ingredient

- 1 can of tuna in water, drained
- 1 ripe avocado, peeled, pitted, and diced
- 1 tablespoon of lemon juice
- 1 tablespoon of olive oil
- 1 tablespoon of finely chopped red onion
- 1 teaspoon of Dijon mustard
- Salt and pepper to taste
- 8 large lettuce leaves (such as romaine or butter lettuce)

Instructions

1. In a medium bowl, combine the drained tuna, diced avocado, lemon juice, olive oil, chopped red onion, and Dijon mustard.
2. Gently mix the ingredients together until well combined, being careful not to mash the avocado too much.
3. Season the mixture with salt and pepper to taste.
4. Lay out the lettuce leaves on a clean surface.
5. Spoon the tuna and avocado mixture evenly onto the center of each lettuce leaf.
6. Fold the sides of the lettuce leaves over the filling and roll them up to form wraps.

7. Serve immediately or refrigerate until ready to eat.

Nutritional Information

- Calories: 150 per wrap
- Protein: 10g
- Carbohydrates: 5g
- Fat: 10g
- Fiber: 3g
- Sodium: 250mg

Serving Size

- Makes 4 servings

Cooking Time

- Preparation: 15 minutes

Chicken and Sweet Potato Soup

Ingredients:

- 2 boneless, skinless chicken breasts
- 2 large sweet potatoes, peeled and diced
- 1 large carrot, peeled and diced
- 1 celery stalk, diced
- 1 small onion, finely chopped
- 2 cloves garlic, minced
- 4 cups low-sodium chicken broth
- 1 cup water
- 1 teaspoon dried thyme
- 1 teaspoon dried rosemary
- Salt and pepper to taste
- 2 tablespoons olive oil

Instructions:

1. In a large pot, heat the olive oil over medium heat.
2. Add the chopped onion and garlic, sautéing until the onion becomes translucent.
3. Add the diced carrot and celery, cooking for another 5 minutes until they start to soften.

4. Add the chicken breasts to the pot and pour in the chicken broth and water.

5. Stir in the dried thyme, rosemary, salt, and pepper.

6. Bring the mixture to a boil, then reduce the heat to a simmer.

7. Cover the pot and let it cook for 20 minutes.

8. Remove the chicken breasts from the pot and shred them using two forks.

9. Return the shredded chicken to the pot and add the diced sweet potatoes.

10. Continue to simmer for another 15 minutes, or until the sweet potatoes are tender.

11. Adjust seasoning with salt and pepper if necessary.

12. Serve hot, garnished with fresh herbs if desired.

Nutritional Information:

- Calories: 250 per serving
- Protein: 20 grams
- Carbohydrates: 25 grams
- Fat: 8 grams
- Sodium: 300 milligrams

Serving Size:

- Serves 4

Cooking Time:

- Total: 50 minutes
  - Preparation: 10 minutes
  - Cooking: 40 minutes

Turkey and Spinach Salad

Ingredient:

- 2 cups fresh spinach leaves, washed and dried
- 1 cup cooked turkey breast, sliced
- 1/2 cup sliced cucumbers
- 1/4 cup shredded carrots
- 1/4 cup chopped red bell pepper
- 2 tablespoons olive oil
- 1 tablespoon apple cider vinegar
- 1 teaspoon Dijon mustard
- Salt and pepper to taste

Instructions:

1. In a large salad bowl, combine the spinach leaves, sliced turkey breast, cucumbers, shredded carrots, and chopped red bell pepper.
2. In a small bowl, whisk together the olive oil, apple cider vinegar, Dijon mustard, salt, and pepper until well combined.
3. Pour the dressing over the salad and toss gently to coat all the ingredients evenly.
4. Serve immediately or chill in the refrigerator for up to an hour before serving.

Nutritional Information (per serving):

- Calories: 250
- Protein: 20g
- Carbohydrates: 6g
- Fiber: 2g
- Fat: 16g
- Sodium: 150mg

Serving Size: 2 servings

Cooking Time: 15 minutes

Rice Noodle and Vegetable Soup

Ingredient:

- 2 cups fresh spinach leaves, washed and dried
- 1 cup cooked turkey breast, sliced
- 1/2 cup sliced cucumbers
- 1/4 cup shredded carrots
- 1/4 cup chopped red bell pepper
- 2 tablespoons olive oil
- 1 tablespoon apple cider vinegar
- 1 teaspoon Dijon mustard
- Salt and pepper to taste

Instructions:

1. In a large salad bowl, combine the spinach leaves, sliced turkey breast, cucumbers, shredded carrots, and chopped red bell pepper.
2. In a small bowl, whisk together the olive oil, apple cider vinegar, Dijon mustard, salt, and pepper until well combined.
3. Pour the dressing over the salad and toss gently to coat all the ingredients evenly.
4. Serve immediately or chill in the refrigerator for up to an hour before serving.

Nutritional Information (per serving):

- Calories: 250
- Protein: 20g
- Carbohydrates: 6g
- Fiber: 2g
- Fat: 16g
- Sodium: 150mg

Serving Size: 2 servings

Cooking Time: 15 minutes

Lemon Herb Chicken with Quinoa

Ingredient:

- 2 boneless, skinless chicken breasts
- 1 cup quinoa, rinsed
- 2 cups low-sodium chicken broth
- 2 tablespoons olive oil
- 1 lemon, juiced and zested
- 2 garlic cloves, minced
- 1 teaspoon dried oregano
- 1 teaspoon dried thyme
- Salt and pepper to taste
- Fresh parsley for garnish

Instructions:

1. Preheat the oven to 375°F (190°C).
2. In a medium saucepan, bring the chicken broth to a boil. Add the quinoa, reduce heat to low, cover, and simmer for about 15 minutes, or until the quinoa is cooked and the liquid is absorbed. Fluff with a fork.

3. While the quinoa is cooking, heat 1 tablespoon of olive oil in a skillet over medium-high heat. Season the chicken breasts with salt, pepper, oregano, and thyme.

4. Add the chicken breasts to the skillet and cook for about 5 minutes on each side, or until golden brown.

5. Transfer the chicken to a baking dish. In a small bowl, mix the lemon juice, lemon zest, remaining olive oil, and minced garlic. Pour this mixture over the chicken.

6. Bake the chicken in the preheated oven for 20-25 minutes, or until the chicken is cooked through and no longer pink in the center.

7. Serve the chicken over the cooked quinoa, garnished with fresh parsley.

Nutritional Information:

- Calories: 350 per serving
- Protein: 25g
- Carbohydrates: 30g
- Fat: 15g
- Fiber: 4g
- Sodium: 150mg

Serving Size:

- Serves 2

Cooking Time:

- Total: 45 minutes

Cottage Cheese and Cucumber Salad

Ingredients:

- 1 cup cottage cheese
- 1 medium cucumber, diced
- 1 tablespoon fresh dill, chopped
- 1 tablespoon fresh parsley, chopped
- 1 tablespoon lemon juice
- Salt and pepper to taste

Instructions:

1. In a large bowl, combine the cottage cheese, diced cucumber, dill, and parsley.
2. Add the lemon juice and mix well.
3. Season with salt and pepper to taste.
4. Serve immediately or refrigerate for up to 1 hour to allow the flavors to meld.

Nutritional Information:

- Calories: 150
- Protein: 12g
- Carbohydrates: 8g

- Fat: 8g
- Fiber: 1g
- Sodium: 400mg

Serving Size:

- Serves 2

Cooking Time:

- Preparation: 10 minutes
- Total: 10 minutes

Beef and Rice Stuffed Peppers

Ingredients:

- 4 bell peppers (any color)
- 1 pound ground beef
- 1 cup cooked white rice
- 1 small onion, finely chopped
- 2 cloves garlic, minced
- 1 cup tomato sauce
- 1 teaspoon dried oregano
- 1 teaspoon dried basil
- Salt and pepper to taste
- 1 tablespoon olive oil
- 1 cup shredded mozzarella cheese (optional)

Instructions:

1. Preheat the oven to 375°F (190°C).
2. Cut the tops off the bell peppers and remove the seeds and membranes. Rinse well and set aside.
3. In a large skillet, heat the olive oil over medium heat. Add the chopped onion and garlic, sautéing until softened and fragrant, about 3-4 minutes.

4. Add the ground beef to the skillet and cook until browned, breaking it up with a spoon as it cooks, about 7-10 minutes. Drain any excess fat.

5. Stir in the cooked rice, tomato sauce, oregano, basil, salt, and pepper. Cook for an additional 5 minutes, allowing the flavors to meld together.

6. Stuff each bell pepper with the beef and rice mixture, packing it in firmly. Place the stuffed peppers upright in a baking dish.

7. Cover the dish with aluminum foil and bake in the preheated oven for 35 minutes.

8. If using, sprinkle the shredded mozzarella cheese over the tops of the peppers and bake uncovered for an additional 10 minutes, or until the cheese is melted and bubbly.

9. Remove from the oven and let cool slightly before serving.

Nutritional Information:

- Calories: 350 per stuffed pepper
- Protein: 20g
- Carbohydrates: 30g
- Fat: 15g
- Fiber: 5g
- Sodium: 600mg

Serving Size:

- 1 stuffed pepper

Cooking Time:

- Total: 1 hour

Roasted Beet and Carrot Salad

Ingredients:

- 2 medium beets, peeled and cut into wedges
- 3 large carrots, peeled and sliced
- 2 tablespoons olive oil
- Salt to taste
- 1 tablespoon lemon juice
- 1 teaspoon honey
- 1/2 cup feta cheese, crumbled
- 1/4 cup chopped fresh parsley

Instructions:

1. Preheat the oven to 400°F (200°C).
2. In a large bowl, toss the beet wedges and carrot slices with 1 tablespoon of olive oil and a pinch of salt.
3. Spread the vegetables on a baking sheet in a single layer.
4. Roast in the preheated oven for 25-30 minutes, or until tender and lightly browned.
5. In a small bowl, whisk together the remaining tablespoon of olive oil, lemon juice, and honey.
6. Once the vegetables are roasted, transfer them to a serving bowl.

7. Drizzle the lemon juice mixture over the vegetables and toss to combine.

8. Sprinkle the crumbled feta cheese and chopped parsley on top.

9. Serve immediately or chill in the refrigerator for a cool, refreshing salad.

Nutritional Information:

- Calories: 180
- Protein: 4g
- Carbohydrates: 18g
- Fat: 10g
- Fiber: 5g
- Sodium: 220mg

Serving Size:

- Serves 4

Cooking Time:

- Preparation: 15 minutes
- Cooking: 30 minutes

Chapter 3: Dinner Recipes

Baked Lemon Herb Fish

Ingredient:

- 4 white fish fillets (such as cod or tilapia)
- 2 lemons (one sliced, one juiced)
- 2 tablespoons olive oil
- 2 cloves garlic, minced
- 1 teaspoon dried thyme
- 1 teaspoon dried parsley
- 1/2 teaspoon salt
- 1/4 teaspoon black pepper
- Fresh parsley for garnish (optional)

Instructions:

1. Preheat the oven to 375°F (190°C).
2. Place the fish fillets in a baking dish.
3. In a small bowl, mix the lemon juice, olive oil, minced garlic, dried thyme, dried parsley, salt, and black pepper.
4. Pour the lemon herb mixture over the fish fillets, ensuring they are evenly coated.

5. Arrange lemon slices on top of the fish.

6. Bake in the preheated oven for 20-25 minutes, or until the fish is opaque and flakes easily with a fork.

7. Garnish with fresh parsley before serving, if desired.

Nutritional Information:

- Calories: 210 per serving
- Protein: 25g
- Fat: 10g
- Carbohydrates: 4g
- Fiber: 1g
- Sodium: 300mg

Serving Size:

- Serves 4

Cooking Time:

- Total time: 30 minutes

Chicken and Rice Casserole

Ingredients:

- 1 pound boneless, skinless chicken breasts, cubed
- 1 cup white rice, uncooked
- 2 cups low-sodium chicken broth
- 1 cup carrots, diced
- 1 cup green beans, cut into 1-inch pieces
- 1 small onion, finely chopped
- 2 cloves garlic, minced
- 1 cup low-fat milk
- 1 cup grated cheddar cheese
- 2 tablespoons olive oil
- 1 teaspoon dried thyme
- 1 teaspoon dried parsley
- Salt and pepper to taste

Instructions:

1. Preheat the oven to 375°F (190°C).
2. Heat the olive oil in a large skillet over medium heat.
3. Add the chicken, onion, and garlic to the skillet. Cook until the chicken is browned and the onion is translucent, about 5-7 minutes.

4. In a large mixing bowl, combine the uncooked rice, carrots, green beans, and the cooked chicken mixture.

5. Add the chicken broth, milk, thyme, parsley, salt, and pepper to the bowl. Stir until well combined.

6. Transfer the mixture to a greased 9x13-inch baking dish.

7. Cover the dish with aluminum foil and bake in the preheated oven for 45 minutes.

8. Remove the foil, sprinkle the cheddar cheese over the top, and return to the oven. Bake uncovered for an additional 10-15 minutes, or until the cheese is melted and bubbly.

9. Allow the casserole to cool for a few minutes before serving.

Nutritional Information:

- Calories: 350 per serving
- Protein: 30g
- Carbohydrates: 30g
- Fat: 12g
- Fiber: 4g
- Sodium: 350mg

Serving Size:

- Serves 6

Cooking Time:

- Total: 1 hour

Ingredients:

- 1 lb lean beef sirloin, thinly sliced
- 2 cups broccoli florets
- 1 red bell pepper, sliced
- 1 yellow bell pepper, sliced
- 1 medium carrot, julienned
- 2 cloves garlic, minced
- 1 inch fresh ginger, grated
- 2 tablespoons olive oil
- 1 tablespoon low-sodium soy sauce
- 1 tablespoon rice vinegar
- 1 tablespoon cornstarch mixed with 2 tablespoons water (for thickening)
- Salt and pepper to taste

Instructions:

1. Heat 1 tablespoon of olive oil in a large skillet or wok over medium-high heat.
2. Add the sliced beef to the skillet and season with salt and pepper. Stir-fry until browned and cooked through, about 5-7 minutes. Remove the beef from the skillet and set aside.

3. In the same skillet, add the remaining tablespoon of olive oil.

4. Add the garlic and ginger, sautéing for about 1 minute until fragrant.

5. Add the broccoli, bell peppers, and carrot to the skillet. Stir-fry for about 5-7 minutes until the vegetables are tender-crisp.

6. Return the beef to the skillet and stir in the low-sodium soy sauce and rice vinegar.

7. Pour the cornstarch mixture into the skillet, stirring constantly until the sauce thickens, about 1-2 minutes.

8. Adjust seasoning with additional salt and pepper if needed.

9. Serve the stir-fry hot over a bed of steamed white rice or quinoa.

Nutritional Information (per serving):

- Calories: 350
- Protein: 30g
- Carbohydrates: 20g
- Fat: 15g
- Sodium: 250mg
- Fiber: 5g

Serving Size:

- 4 servings

Cooking Time:

- Preparation Time: 10 minutes
- Cooking Time: 20 minutes
- Total Time: 30 minutes

Quinoa and Turkey Meatloaf

Ingredient

1 cup cooked quinoa

1 lb ground turkey

1 small onion, finely chopped

1 garlic clove, minced

1 egg, lightly beaten

1/4 cup finely chopped parsley

1 tsp dried thyme

1/2 tsp salt

1/4 tsp black pepper

1/2 cup tomato sauce

Instructions

1. Preheat the oven to 375°F (190°C). Grease a loaf pan with a small amount of oil or line it with parchment paper.
2. In a large mixing bowl, combine the cooked quinoa, ground turkey, chopped onion, minced garlic, beaten egg, chopped parsley, dried thyme, salt, and black pepper. Mix until all ingredients are well incorporated.

3. Transfer the mixture into the prepared loaf pan and press it down evenly. Pour the tomato sauce over the top of the meatloaf, spreading it out evenly with a spatula.

4. Bake in the preheated oven for 45-50 minutes or until the meatloaf is cooked through and the internal temperature reaches 165°F (74°C).

5. Remove from the oven and let it rest for 10 minutes before slicing and serving.

Nutritional Information

Calories: 280
Protein: 25g
Carbohydrates: 18g
Fat: 10g
Fiber: 3g

Serving Size

Serves 4

Cooking Time

Preparation: 20 minutes
Cooking: 50 minutes

Stuffed Bell Peppers with Rice and Beef

Ingredients:

- 4 large bell peppers (any color)
- 1 pound ground beef (preferably lean)
- 1 cup cooked white rice
- 1 small onion, finely chopped
- 2 cloves garlic, minced
- 1 cup tomato sauce (nickel-free)
- 1 teaspoon dried oregano
- 1 teaspoon dried basil
- Salt and pepper to taste
- 1 tablespoon olive oil
- 1 cup shredded mozzarella cheese (optional)

Instructions:

1. Preheat the oven to 375°F (190°C).
2. Cut the tops off the bell peppers and remove the seeds and membranes. Set aside.
3. In a large skillet, heat the olive oil over medium heat. Add the chopped onion and garlic, sautéing until softened and fragrant, about 3-4 minutes.

4. Add the ground beef to the skillet, breaking it apart with a spoon, and cook until browned and fully cooked through. Drain any excess fat.

5. Stir in the cooked rice, tomato sauce, dried oregano, dried basil, salt, and pepper. Cook for an additional 5 minutes, allowing the flavors to meld together.

6. Stuff each bell pepper with the beef and rice mixture, packing it in firmly.

7. Place the stuffed peppers upright in a baking dish. Cover with aluminum foil and bake for 30 minutes.

8. If using mozzarella cheese, remove the foil after 30 minutes, sprinkle the cheese on top of the peppers, and bake uncovered for an additional 10 minutes, until the cheese is melted and bubbly.

9. Remove from the oven and let the peppers cool for a few minutes before serving.

Nutritional Information:

- Calories: 350 per serving
- Protein: 25g
- Carbohydrates: 20g
- Fat: 18g
- Fiber: 3g
- Sodium: 600mg

Serving Size:

- Serves 4

Cooking Time:

- Total: 50 minutes

Herb-Crusted Pork Tenderloin

Ingredient

- 1 pound pork tenderloin
- 2 tablespoons olive oil
- 1 tablespoon fresh rosemary, chopped
- 1 tablespoon fresh thyme, chopped
- 1 tablespoon fresh parsley, chopped
- 2 cloves garlic, minced
- 1 teaspoon salt
- 1/2 teaspoon black pepper

Instructions

1. Preheat your oven to 375°F (190°C).
2. In a small bowl, combine the rosemary, thyme, parsley, garlic, salt, and black pepper.
3. Rub the pork tenderloin with olive oil, then coat it evenly with the herb mixture.
4. Place the pork tenderloin on a baking sheet lined with parchment paper.
5. Roast in the preheated oven for 25-30 minutes, or until the internal temperature reaches 145°F (63°C).
6. Remove from the oven and let rest for 5 minutes before slicing.

Nutritional Information

- Calories: 250 per serving
- Protein: 28g
- Fat: 14g
- Carbohydrates: 1g
- Fiber: 0g
- Sodium: 520mg

Serving Size

- 4 servings

Cooking Time

- Total time: 40 minutes

Rice and Chicken Pilaf

Ingredients

- 1 cup long-grain white rice
- 2 cups low-sodium chicken broth
- 1 pound boneless, skinless chicken breasts, diced
- 1 tablespoon olive oil
- 1 small onion, finely chopped
- 1 carrot, finely chopped
- 1 celery stalk, finely chopped
- 2 cloves garlic, minced
- 1 teaspoon dried thyme
- Salt and pepper to taste
- Fresh parsley, chopped (optional, for garnish)

Instructions

1. In a large skillet, heat the olive oil over medium heat. Add the diced chicken and cook until browned and cooked through, about 5-7 minutes. Remove the chicken from the skillet and set aside.
2. In the same skillet, add the chopped onion, carrot, and celery. Cook until the vegetables are tender, about 5 minutes.

3. Add the minced garlic and dried thyme to the skillet and cook for an additional minute, until fragrant.

4. Stir in the rice and cook for 1-2 minutes, until the rice is lightly toasted.

5. Pour in the low-sodium chicken broth and bring to a boil.

6. Reduce the heat to low, cover, and simmer for 15-20 minutes, or until the rice is cooked and the liquid is absorbed.

7. Return the cooked chicken to the skillet and stir to combine. Season with salt and pepper to taste.

8. Garnish with chopped parsley, if desired, before serving.

Nutritional Information

- Calories: 350 per serving
- Protein: 25 grams
- Carbohydrates: 40 grams
- Fat: 10 grams
- Sodium: 300 milligrams

Serving Size

- Serves 4

Cooking Time

- 35 minutes

Shrimp and Vegetable Skewers

Ingredients:

- 1 lb large shrimp, peeled and deveined
- 1 red bell pepper, cut into 1-inch pieces
- 1 yellow bell pepper, cut into 1-inch pieces
- 1 zucchini, cut into 1/2-inch rounds
- 1 red onion, cut into wedges
- 2 tbsp olive oil
- 2 tbsp lemon juice
- 2 cloves garlic, minced
- 1 tsp dried oregano
- Salt and pepper to taste

Instructions:

1. Preheat the grill to medium-high heat.
2. In a large bowl, combine the olive oil, lemon juice, garlic, oregano, salt, and pepper. Mix well.
3. Add the shrimp and vegetables to the bowl, tossing to coat them evenly with the marinade. Let sit for 10-15 minutes.
4. Thread the shrimp and vegetables onto skewers, alternating pieces for variety.

5. Place the skewers on the grill and cook for 2-3 minutes per side, or until the shrimp are opaque and the vegetables are tender.

6. Remove from the grill and serve immediately.

Nutritional Information (per serving):

- Calories: 210
- Protein: 22g
- Carbohydrates: 8g
- Dietary Fiber: 2g
- Sugars: 3g
- Fat: 10g
- Saturated Fat: 1.5g
- Cholesterol: 145mg
- Sodium: 300mg

Serving Size: 4 skewers

Cooking Time: 20 minutes

Sweet and Sour Chicken

Ingredients:

- 1 lb chicken breast, cut into bite-sized pieces
- 1/2 cup pineapple juice (low nickel)
- 1/4 cup apple cider vinegar
- 1/4 cup low-sodium soy sauce (ensure it is nickel-free)
- 2 tbsp brown sugar
- 1 tbsp cornstarch
- 1 bell pepper, cut into strips
- 1 onion, cut into wedges
- 1 cup pineapple chunks (low nickel)
- 2 cloves garlic, minced
- 1 tbsp olive oil
- Salt and pepper to taste

Instructions:

1. In a bowl, mix the pineapple juice, apple cider vinegar, soy sauce, and brown sugar. Set aside.

2. In a separate bowl, dissolve the cornstarch in a small amount of cold water to create a slurry.

3. Season the chicken pieces with salt and pepper.

4. Heat olive oil in a large skillet over medium-high heat. Add the chicken and cook until browned and fully cooked, about 5-7 minutes.

5. Remove the chicken from the skillet and set aside.

6. In the same skillet, add the garlic, bell pepper, and onion. Sauté for 3-4 minutes until the vegetables are tender.

7. Return the chicken to the skillet and add the pineapple chunks.

8. Pour the pineapple juice mixture over the chicken and vegetables.

9. Stir in the cornstarch slurry to thicken the sauce. Cook for an additional 2-3 minutes until the sauce has thickened.

10. Adjust seasoning with salt and pepper as needed.

11. Serve hot, preferably with a side of steamed white rice or a low nickel grain.

Nutritional Information:

- Calories: 350 per serving
- Protein: 25g
- Carbohydrates: 30g
- Fat: 12g
- Fiber: 3g
- Sodium: 450mg
- Sugars: 15g

Serving Size:

- Serves 4

Cooking Time:

- Total time: 30 minutes

Vegetable and Rice Stew

Ingredient

- 1 cup of white rice
- 2 cups of low-sodium vegetable broth
- 1 cup of water
- 1 medium carrot, diced
- 1 zucchini, diced
- 1 cup of green beans, trimmed and cut into pieces
- 1 red bell pepper, diced
- 1 small onion, finely chopped
- 2 cloves of garlic, minced
- 1 tablespoon of olive oil
- 1 teaspoon of dried thyme
- 1 teaspoon of dried oregano
- Salt and pepper to taste

Instructions

1. Rinse the white rice under cold water until the water runs clear. Set aside.

2. In a large pot, heat the olive oil over medium heat. Add the chopped onion and minced garlic, and sauté until the onion becomes translucent.

3. Add the diced carrot, zucchini, green beans, and red bell pepper to the pot. Cook for about 5 minutes, stirring occasionally, until the vegetables start to soften.

4. Stir in the rinsed white rice, ensuring it is well mixed with the vegetables.

5. Pour in the low-sodium vegetable broth and water, then add the dried thyme and oregano. Stir to combine.

6. Bring the mixture to a boil, then reduce the heat to low. Cover the pot and simmer for about 20 minutes, or until the rice is cooked and the vegetables are tender.

7. Season with salt and pepper to taste. If the stew is too thick, you can add a bit more water to reach the desired consistency.

8. Serve hot, garnished with fresh herbs if desired.

Nutritional Information

- Calories: 180 per serving
- Carbohydrates: 32g
- Protein: 4g
- Fat: 5g
- Fiber: 3g
- Sodium: 200mg
- Potassium: 450mg

Serving Size

- Serves 4

Cooking Time

- 35 minutes

Chapter 4: Snacks and Sides

Safe and Tasty Snack Options

Baked Apple Chips

- **Ingredient**: Apples, cinnamon
- **Instructions**: Slice apples thinly and sprinkle with cinnamon. Bake at 225°F for 2 hours, flipping halfway.
- **Nutritional Information**: 95 calories per serving, 0g fat, 25g carbohydrates, 4g fiber, 0g protein
- **Serving Size**: 1 medium apple
- **Cooking Time**: 2 hours

Carrot and Cucumber Sticks with Hummus

- **Ingredient**: Carrots, cucumbers, homemade hummus (chickpeas, tahini, lemon juice, garlic, olive oil)
- **Instructions**: Cut carrots and cucumbers into sticks. Blend chickpeas, tahini, lemon juice, garlic, and olive oil to make hummus.

- **Nutritional Information**: 150 calories per serving, 8g fat, 16g
carbohydrates, 6g fiber, 5g protein
- **Serving Size**: 1 cup of vegetables with 1/4 cup hummus
- **Cooking Time**: 15 minutes

Cinnamon-Sugar Popcorn

- **Ingredient**: Popcorn kernels, coconut oil, cinnamon, sugar
- **Instructions**: Pop kernels in coconut oil, then sprinkle with a
mixture of cinnamon and sugar.
- **Nutritional Information**: 100 calories per serving, 4.5g fat,
15g carbohydrates, 3g fiber, 2g protein
- **Serving Size**: 2 cups
- **Cooking Time**: 10 minutes

Rice Crackers with Avocado Dip

- **Ingredient**: Rice crackers, avocados, lime juice, garlic powder,
salt
- **Instructions**: Mash avocados with lime juice, garlic powder, and
salt. Serve with rice crackers.
- **Nutritional Information**: 180 calories per serving, 12g fat, 18g
carbohydrates, 5g fiber, 2g protein
- **Serving Size**: 10 crackers with 1/2 avocado dip
- **Cooking Time**: 10 minutes

Greek Yogurt with Honey and Blueberries

- **Ingredient**: Greek yogurt, honey, blueberries
- **Instructions**: Mix Greek yogurt with honey and top with fresh blueberries.
- **Nutritional Information**: 150 calories per serving, 2g fat, 25g carbohydrates, 3g fiber, 10g protein
- **Serving Size**: 1 cup
- **Cooking Time**: 5 minutes

Homemade Granola Bars

- **Ingredient**: Oats, honey, dried cranberries, sunflower seeds, coconut oil
- **Instructions**: Mix ingredients and press into a baking dish. Bake at 325°F for 25 minutes.
- **Nutritional Information**: 200 calories per serving, 8g fat, 30g carbohydrates, 4g fiber, 5g protein
- **Serving Size**: 1 bar
- **Cooking Time**: 30 minutes

Vegetable Spring Rolls

- **Ingredient**: Rice paper, lettuce, carrots, cucumbers, bell peppers, mint leaves, low-nickel dipping sauce

- **Instructions**: Soak rice paper and fill with vegetables and mint leaves. Roll tightly and serve with dipping sauce.
- **Nutritional Information**: 120 calories per serving, 2g fat, 25g carbohydrates, 5g fiber, 3g protein
- **Serving Size**: 2 rolls
- **Cooking Time**: 20 minutes

Roasted Chickpeas

- **Ingredient**: Canned chickpeas, olive oil, paprika, garlic powder, salt
- **Instructions**: Toss chickpeas with olive oil and spices. Roast at 400°F for 30 minutes.
- **Nutritional Information**: 150 calories per serving, 5g fat, 20g carbohydrates, 6g fiber, 7g protein
- **Serving Size**: 1/2 cup
- **Cooking Time**: 35 minutes

Fruit and Nut Mix

- **Ingredient**: Dried apricots, raisins, sunflower seeds, pumpkin seeds
- **Instructions**: Combine all ingredients in a bowl.
- **Nutritional Information**: 200 calories per serving, 9g fat, 30g carbohydrates, 5g fiber, 6g protein
- **Serving Size**: 1/2 cup
- **Cooking Time**: 5 minutes

Zucchini Chips

- **Ingredient**: Zucchini, olive oil, sea salt
- **Instructions**: Slice zucchini thinly, toss with olive oil and sea salt. Bake at 225°F for 2 hours, flipping halfway.
- **Nutritional Information**: 80 calories per serving, 3g fat, 12g carbohydrates, 2g fiber, 2g protein
- **Serving Size**: 1 cup
- **Cooking Time**: 2 hours

Roasted Sweet Potato Wedges

Ingredients:
- 2 large sweet potatoes
- 2 tablespoons olive oil
- 1 teaspoon paprika
- 1/2 teaspoon garlic powder
- Salt and pepper to taste

Instructions:
1. Preheat oven to 400°F (200°C).
2. Peel and cut sweet potatoes into wedges.
3. In a bowl, toss the wedges with olive oil, paprika, garlic powder, salt, and pepper.
4. Spread the wedges on a baking sheet in a single layer.
5. Roast for 25-30 minutes, turning halfway through, until golden and crispy.

Nutritional Information:
Calories: 180
Carbohydrates: 30g

Protein: 2g

Fat: 7g

Fiber: 4g

Serving Size:

4 servings

Cooking Time:

35 minutes

Cucumber and Dill Salad

Ingredients:

- 2 large cucumbers
- 1/4 cup fresh dill, chopped
- 2 tablespoons apple cider vinegar
- 1 tablespoon olive oil
- Salt and pepper to taste

Instructions:

1. Slice cucumbers thinly and place them in a large bowl.
2. Add chopped dill, apple cider vinegar, and olive oil.
3. Toss to coat evenly.
4. Season with salt and pepper to taste.
5. Refrigerate for at least 30 minutes before serving for best flavor.

Nutritional Information:

Calories: 60

Carbohydrates: 8g

Protein: 1g

Fat: 3g

Fiber: 1g

Serving Size:

4 servings

Cooking Time:

10 minutes (plus 30 minutes refrigeration)

Apple and Celery Salad

Ingredients:

- 2 apples, diced
- 3 celery stalks, diced
- 1/4 cup plain Greek yogurt
- 1 tablespoon lemon juice
- 1 tablespoon honey
- Salt and pepper to taste

Instructions:

1. In a large bowl, combine diced apples and celery.

2. In a separate bowl, mix Greek yogurt, lemon juice, and honey.

3. Pour the dressing over the apple and celery mixture.

4. Toss to coat evenly.

5. Season with salt and pepper to taste.

Nutritional Information:

Calories: 90

Carbohydrates: 18g

Protein: 2g

Fat: 1g

Fiber: 3g

Serving Size:

4 servings

Cooking Time:

15 minutes

Carrot and Ginger Soup

Ingredients:

- 4 large carrots, peeled and chopped
- 1 small onion, chopped
- 1-inch piece of ginger, grated
- 2 cups low-sodium chicken broth
- 1 tablespoon olive oil
- Salt and pepper to taste

Instructions:

1. Heat olive oil in a pot over medium heat.

2. Add chopped onion and cook until soft, about 5 minutes.

3. Add carrots and ginger, cooking for another 5 minutes.

4. Pour in chicken broth and bring to a boil.

5. Reduce heat and simmer until carrots are tender, about 20 minutes.

6. Blend the soup until smooth.

7. Season with salt and pepper to taste.

Nutritional Information:

Calories: 100

Carbohydrates: 20g

Protein: 2g

Fat: 3g

Fiber: 5g

Serving Size:

4 servings

Cooking Time:

35 minutes

Zucchini Fritters

Ingredients:

- 2 medium zucchinis, grated
- 1 egg, beaten
- 1/4 cup flour
- 2 tablespoons grated Parmesan cheese
- 1 teaspoon garlic powder
- Salt and pepper to taste
- Olive oil for frying

Instructions:

1. Grate zucchinis and squeeze out excess moisture using a clean towel.
2. In a bowl, mix grated zucchini, beaten egg, flour, Parmesan cheese, garlic powder, salt, and pepper.
3. Heat olive oil in a skillet over medium heat.
4. Drop spoonfuls of the mixture into the skillet and flatten slightly.
5. Fry until golden brown on both sides, about 3-4 minutes per side.
6. Drain on paper towels before serving.

Nutritional Information:

Calories: 150
Carbohydrates: 10g
Protein: 5g
Fat: 10g
Fiber: 2g

Serving Size:

4 servings

Cooking Time:

20 minutes

Chapter 5: Desserts

Low Nickel Sweet Treats

Vanilla Rice Pudding

Ingredients:
- 1 cup white rice
- 4 cups whole milk
- 1/2 cup granulated sugar
- 1 vanilla bean, split and seeds scraped
- 1/4 teaspoon salt
- 1/4 teaspoon ground cinnamon (optional)

Instructions:
1. In a large saucepan, combine the rice, milk, sugar, vanilla bean and seeds, and salt.
2. Bring the mixture to a boil over medium heat, stirring frequently.
3. Reduce the heat to low and simmer, stirring occasionally, until the rice is tender and the mixture has thickened, about 45 minutes.

4. Remove from heat and let it cool slightly. Remove the vanilla bean pod.

5. Sprinkle with ground cinnamon if desired before serving.

Nutritional Information:
- Calories: 250 per serving
- Carbohydrates: 50g
- Protein: 6g
- Fat: 5g
- Sodium: 100mg

Serving Size:
- Serves 4

Cooking Time:
- 50 minutes

Apple Oatmeal Cookies

Ingredients:
- 1 cup rolled oats
- 1/2 cup white rice flour
- 1/2 teaspoon baking soda
- 1/4 teaspoon salt
- 1/2 cup unsalted butter, softened
- 1/2 cup granulated sugar

- 1/4 cup light brown sugar, packed
- 1 large egg
- 1 teaspoon vanilla extract
- 1/2 cup finely chopped apple (peeled)

Instructions:

1. Preheat your oven to 350°F (175°C) and line a baking sheet with parchment paper.
2. In a medium bowl, mix together the oats, rice flour, baking soda, and salt.
3. In a separate bowl, cream together the butter, granulated sugar, and brown sugar until light and fluffy.
4. Beat in the egg and vanilla extract until well combined.
5. Gradually add the dry ingredients to the wet ingredients, mixing until just combined.
6. Fold in the chopped apple.
7. Drop spoonfuls of dough onto the prepared baking sheet.
8. Bake for 12-15 minutes, or until the edges are golden brown.
9. Let the cookies cool on the baking sheet for a few minutes before transferring to a wire rack to cool completely.

Nutritional Information:
- Calories: 150 per cookie
- Carbohydrates: 20g
- Protein: 2g
- Fat: 7g
- Sodium: 80mg

Serving Size:
- Makes about 24 cookies

Cooking Time:
- 20 minutes

Lemon Sorbet

Ingredients:
- 1 cup water
- 1 cup granulated sugar
- 1 cup freshly squeezed lemon juice (about 4-6 lemons)
- 1 tablespoon lemon zest

Instructions:
1. In a small saucepan, combine the water and sugar. Heat over medium heat, stirring until the sugar is dissolved.
2. Remove from heat and let the syrup cool completely.
3. Stir in the lemon juice and lemon zest.
4. Pour the mixture into an ice cream maker and freeze according to the manufacturer's instructions.
5. Transfer the sorbet to an airtight container and freeze for at least 2 hours, or until firm.

Nutritional Information:

- Calories: 100 per serving
- Carbohydrates: 25g
- Protein: 0g
- Fat: 0g
- Sodium: 5mg

Serving Size:
- Serves 6

Cooking Time:
- 10 minutes (plus freezing time)

Apple Cinnamon Crumble

Ingredients:
- 4 large apples, peeled and sliced
- 1 teaspoon ground cinnamon
- 1 tablespoon lemon juice
- 1/2 cup oats (certified low nickel)
- 1/4 cup brown sugar
- 1/4 cup butter, melted

Instructions:
1. Preheat the oven to 350°F (175°C).
2. In a bowl, toss the apple slices with cinnamon and lemon juice.
3. Spread the apples evenly in a baking dish.
4. In another bowl, mix the oats, brown sugar, and melted butter until crumbly.
5. Sprinkle the oat mixture over the apples.
6. Bake for 30-35 minutes, until the apples are tender and the topping is golden brown.

Nutritional Information:

- Calories: 180 per serving
- Carbohydrates: 28g
- Protein: 2g
- Fat: 7g
- Fiber: 4g

Serving Size:
- Serves 6

Cooking Time:
- 40 minutes total

Berry Yogurt Parfait

Ingredients:
- 2 cups Greek yogurt (plain, low-fat)
- 1 cup strawberries, hulled and sliced
- 1 cup blueberries
- 1 tablespoon honey
- 1 teaspoon vanilla extract
- 1/2 cup granola (certified low nickel)

Instructions:
1. In a bowl, mix the yogurt, honey, and vanilla extract.
2. In serving glasses, layer yogurt, strawberries, and blueberries.
3. Repeat the layers until the glasses are full.

4. Top with granola just before serving to maintain crunch.

Nutritional Information:
- Calories: 200 per serving
- Carbohydrates: 30g
- Protein: 10g
- Fat: 5g
- Fiber: 3g

Serving Size:
- Serves 4

Cooking Time:
- 10 minutes total

Lemon Sorbet

Ingredients:
- 1 cup fresh lemon juice (about 4-5 lemons)
- 1 cup water
- 3/4 cup sugar
- 1 tablespoon lemon zest

Instructions:
1. In a saucepan, combine water and sugar. Heat until sugar dissolves.

2. Remove from heat and stir in lemon juice and zest.

3. Pour the mixture into a shallow dish and freeze for 3 hours, stirring every 30 minutes to break up ice crystals.

Nutritional Information:

- Calories: 100 per serving

- Carbohydrates: 26g

- Protein: 0g

- Fat: 0g

- Fiber: 0g

Serving Size:

- Serves 6

Cooking Time:

- 3 hours 10 minutes total

Conclusion

The "Low Nickel Diet Cookbook 2024" serves as an indispensable guide for those navigating the challenges of a low-nickel diet. This cookbook goes beyond merely offering recipes; it provides a comprehensive approach to managing dietary restrictions while still enjoying a wide variety of flavorful and satisfying meals. The thoughtfully curated recipes ensure that individuals with nickel sensitivities can maintain a balanced and nutritious diet without feeling deprived.

Throughout this cookbook, the emphasis has been on creating delicious meals that are easy to prepare and adhere to low-nickel guidelines. From hearty breakfasts and nourishing lunches to delectable dinners and indulgent desserts, each recipe has been meticulously crafted to minimize nickel content while maximizing taste and nutritional value. This careful attention to ingredient selection and preparation methods ensures that every dish supports a healthy lifestyle and meets the specific dietary needs of those with nickel allergies or sensitivities.

One of the standout features of this cookbook is its dedication to providing a variety of options that cater to different tastes and preferences. Whether you prefer savory dishes, sweet treats, or something in between, the "Low Nickel Diet Cookbook 2024" offers a wide range of choices. This diversity helps to prevent meal fatigue and keeps your diet interesting and enjoyable, encouraging long-term adherence to dietary restrictions.

In addition to the wealth of recipes, this cookbook also includes valuable educational content. Readers will find detailed explanations of what a low-nickel diet entails, the importance of avoiding high-nickel foods, and practical tips for managing nickel intake. This information empowers individuals to make informed decisions about their diet and health, fostering a greater sense of control and confidence in their ability to manage nickel sensitivity.

Meal planning and preparation are further simplified with the inclusion of weekly meal plans and grocery lists. These tools help to streamline the process of shopping for and preparing meals, reducing the stress and time associated with maintaining a low-nickel diet. By providing clear guidance and practical tips, this cookbook ensures that following a low-nickel diet is both manageable and sustainable.

The cookbook also addresses the social and emotional aspects of living with dietary restrictions. By offering delicious and appealing recipes, it helps to mitigate the sense of deprivation that can accompany a restricted diet. This positive approach to food can enhance overall well-being and quality of life, making it easier to embrace and maintain dietary changes.

In conclusion, the "Low Nickel Diet Cookbook 2024" is a valuable resource for anyone managing a nickel sensitivity. It offers a comprehensive and practical approach to low-nickel eating, ensuring that dietary restrictions do not come at the expense of flavor, variety, or enjoyment. With its blend of delicious recipes, educational content, and practical tools, this cookbook is an essential guide for achieving and maintaining a healthy, low-nickel lifestyle.